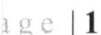

Herbal Hair Remedies from Natures Pharmacy

Table of Contents

Introduction	3
History of Shampoo	5
Harmful Toxins in Commercial Shampoos	9
Avoidable chemicals	10
Friendly Chemicals	14
Benefits of Herbal Shampoo	16
Free of Toxins	17
Fresh Ingredients	17
Custom-made	18
Cost-saving	18
Fun	19
Shampoo Base Ingredients	20
Shampoo Base Recipes	23
Herbal Infusions	25
Herbal Infusion Natural Shampoo Recipes	26
Natural Shampoos with Essential Oil Recipes	35
Hair Spritz Recipes	36
Hair Mask Recipes	37
Oil Treatment Recipes	38
Herbal Hair Rinses	46
Natural Dry Shampoo Recipes	51
Summary	52

Introduction

In today's fast paced, chemically induced life, everyone wants to take a break from it all and visit the country. This is mostly because in the country, we can get back to our roots – to a time of life that was simpler and more wholesome.

We do not really and truly need all of these chemicals in our lives today. One small change you can make yourself is to create your own homemade herbal shampoos. Get back to nature – starting with the roots of your hair!

Having hair that is both strong and beautiful does not equate to using expensive or exotic-sounding hair treatments. Instead, you can use simple, homemade shampoo and conditioner to maintain a healthy head of hair. Homemade herbal shampoos are very easy to make at home and can do wonders in giving your hair plenty of bounce and shine too.

Everyone wants beautiful, shiny hair but most seem to think they have to spend hundreds of dollars at a salon on equally expensive products in order to achieve their desired result. However, this is just not true. Did you know that just by eating a well-balanced diet, drinking plenty of fresh water, and getting at least 8 hours of sleep per day will have a positive effect on both your hair and skin?

Another thing that you can do for your hair is to keep it clean and well-nourished at all times. Our hair is easily affected by humidity, air conditioning, and other air pollution on a daily basis.

In order to properly cleanse your hair you will need to understand that hair care products each have their own specific uses. Shampoo obviously cleans your hair first, but it also invigorates your scalp and removes any dead skin cells. It also loosens up any dirt and residual oils that may be inhabiting your hair.

Conditioners are used to add moisture to your hair – these moisturizers act as a protectant from heat, humidity, and split ends. A rinse is used to thoroughly clean your hair and will remove any prior build-up of other hair products.

History of Shampoo

Humankind has been driven by one simple goal throughout the ages: be attractive to the opposite sex.

Recorded history depicts Egyptian woman covering themselves with colored pigments, bathing in flower petal covered pools, and anointing their bodies in fragrant oils. These oils were made from olives, almonds, sesame, and safflowers and contained fragrances made from steeping wildflowers, herbs, and resins in water.

Romans, Greeks, and Turks took pride in the art of the bathhouse. Scented bath waters laced with salts, powders, and then adding boiled herbs and flowers to the water was discovered to linger on the skin long after leaving the bath.

As time progressed, so did the beauty concoctions of creams, oils, soaps, laundry detergents, and eventually, shampoo.

Human skin has a wonderfully complex system of naturally producing oils and shedding dead layers of skin to promote naturally hydrated skin. The downfall to this system is that it creates a pungent aroma and clothing absorbs the oils from the skin. Dirt and grime build up on the surface of the skin along with the dead layers of skin, adding to the ghastly aroma. This concoction also acts as a breeding ground for bacteria and quickly becomes a health risk to ourselves and to others around us.

Soap contains surfactants that break apart the layers of grease, dirt, grime, and dead skin cells leaving behind cleansed skin ready to start the process all over again.

This process was also used to cleanse hair, as well from grime, dead skin cells, environmental pollutants, and scents picked up from day to day locations. The downsides to using soap was that it stripped away the beneficial oils that keeps hair from becoming dry, brittle, splitting, and unappealing.

Many cultures found that adding naturally occurring oils afterwards helped keep hair from becoming unmanageable. In Indonesia, the use of Coconut oil after washing helped make the hair very silky and moisturized.

India's answer was to use boiled Soapnuts with sun dried Indian Gooseberries and other herbs to make a delightfully scented shampoo that would cleanse the hair and leave it clean and manageable.

Early Europeans took inspiration from many of the newly established trade destinations and the act of massaging the scalp with scented oils and soaps. The word shampoo is taken from the words Champi, Champo, and Capayati, which means to knead, soothe, and press. Later on around the mid 1800's the term became known more for cleansing the hair with soap, than for the act of massage.

In the early 1900's shampoo was made by boiling shaved soap flakes in water and adding fragrant herbs and salts. The earliest recorded commercially made shampoo was advertised around 1914, but what we know as shampoo today, did not come about until the mid-1930's when Proctor and Gamble developed the first non-soap derived surfactant.

Presently there are hundreds of shampoos on the market, many made with modern chemicals and artificial fragrances. These chemicals can cause severe skin reactions and this prompts many consumers to seek a specialist who can diagnose which chemical causes the reaction and help guide them to a brand that does not contain that ingredient. These chemicals are also extremely damaging to the environment when rinsed from your head and down the drain.

There are also manufacturers that do not use the chemicals and seek to use natural ingredients and herbal formulas similar to ancient recipes. With many organic ingredients from around the world formulated to achieve benefits that would never have been possible in the past, modern scientific understanding of these herbal properties, and how best to pair them has been increasingly improving over the years.

However, the only way to ensure proper hair health is to produce your own homemade herbal shampoos, rinses, and treatments.

Creating your own shampoo is a fun and relaxing process that will help you better understand what you are putting in your hair and down the drain.

Harmful Toxins in Commercial Shampoos

Shampoo is a hair product that is used to take away skin particles, dandruff, oil, and dirt from hair. It helps to take care of personal cleanliness and maintain the health of hair. Shampoos are created to specifically clean the scalp of sebum, which is considered as natural oil. Shampoo is used to get rid of the wanted environmental pollutions that have built up on hair over a period of time.

In the history of shampoo, different countries throughout the world used to clean their hair in different ways using different elements that were locally available.

- In Indonesia, the skin and straw of rice used to be burned and turned to ash. This ash has alkaline properties. The ashes were then mixed with water and was used a shampoo.
- In India, soap-nuts, Indian gooseberry, and different kinds of herbs were used as a shampoo.
- Native American people used a variety of North American plant extracts for their shampoo.

Origin of shampoo:

Generally, shampoo is a thick, sticky liquid that is made by combining a surfactant (most often sodium lauryl sulfate) with a co-surfactant (typically Cocamidopropyl) with water.

Mode of action of shampoo:

Shampoo cleans hair by removing sebum. Sebum is an oily element that is secreted through the hair follicles. It is absorbable and protective. It prevents damage of the protein structure of hair. By preventing damage, it has to absorb dirt and scalp flakes. To strip these components shampoo plays a vital role.

Avoidable chemicals

It is very tempting to decide which shampoo to use, based simply on its provocative advertisement. People just buy right off the shelf if they feel emotionally drawn to do so by viewing a products advertisement on television or in a magazine.

However, not many people know that there are many cancers causing ingredients in these commercial hair care products. Many harmful toxic chemicals are hiding under a nice and good name. One should be careful in selecting a shampoo, because not only your hair but also all of your body and organs will be in danger by these harmful components.

Please take a look below at these chemicals and read the label on your shampoo bottle to see how many you can find lurking there:

1. **Sodium Lauryl Sulfate/ Sodium Laureth Sulfate:**

It is a common ingredient in most all shampoos. It is known as SLS. This ingredient helps to create foam and significantly clean the scalp. However, the horrible truth is this ingredient is a cancer-causing ingredient. It is also used as an engine degreaser and is sold in automotive parts store throughout the world. It actually swallows up your scalp's essential oil, which is the necessary element to keeping hair healthy.

2. **Perfume or Fragrance:**

Artificial ingredients are responsible for the sweet-smelling fragrances of shampoo. However, this beautiful "Fragrance" is made from highly toxic fabricated ingredients. These toxic ingredients are responsible for-

- Skin rashes and color changes of skin
- Headaches, and even blackouts
- Damages to the liver, brain, and kidney
- Harmful effects on the central nervous system

3. **Triethanolamine and Diethanolamin:**

These two agents are responsible for cancer and hormonal imbalances. They also cause sensitive scalps, skin sensitivities, and long-term use can create dry and lifeless hair.

4. Propyl, Methyl and Butyl Parben:

These ingredients are used as preservatives. However, they are very much responsible for breast cancer and skin allergies. So they should be ignored when choosing a commercial shampoo.

5. Formaldehyde releases:

Diazolidinyl and imidazolidinyl urea are formaldehyde donors that are used as antimicrobial preservatives. They are very harmful for the skin, as well as the immune system.

6. Shampoo Colors:

We love the colors of shampoos, but it is a bitter truth that all these colors are artificial and can be extremely harmful. They cause cancer, allergies, and even problems with our respiratory organs.

7. PEG (Poly Ethylene Glycol):

The most used ingredient in shampoo is polyethylene glycol. It works as a solvent but it is very harmful because it is also a cancer-creating agent. Therefore, it is a very deadly chemical.

8. Dimethicones and silicones:

Amodimethicone is a silicone-based polymer that creates smooth hair, but they actually prohibit moisture by keeping the scalp dry. This causes hair to fall out, and makes the hair thinner. These polymers are not friendly for any type of hair.

9. Alcohol:

Iso propyl alcohol is a cleanser and it abolishes the oils of the scalp. However, it is also responsible for dryness, hair loss, and hair damage too.

10. 1,4 dioxane:

This byproduct is a common finding in shampoo, even in baby shampoos. Nevertheless, it is very harmful to the brain and central nervous system.

11. Methyl-iso-thiazolinone:

This biocide is used in shampoos for controlling bacterial growth, but in the long run this chemical causes harm in cell-functioning, and also damages the neurons of fetuses.

12. Tocopheryl acetate:

This chemical causes skin irritations, inflammation, and rashes, as well as grave damage to the immune system.

Friendly Chemicals

1. **Glycerin:**

It is a protective chemical, which locks in hair moisture long after shampooing.

2. **Nut and seed oils:**

Jojoba, avocado, and Shea butter are natural moisturizers. They help in removing oily components from the hair and add in shine and moisture to the hair.

3. **Citric acid:**

Sodium citrate helps by maintaining the overall pH balance of shampoo. This balance keeps the hair cuticle healthy and cleans the hair of dirt and oil. This makes hair shiny and smooth.

4. **Vitamins:**

Panthenol, a unique blend of vitamin B1, is used in shampoos to thicken hair and to keep hair healthy and shiny.

Many people regularly clean their hair with shampoo. Most of them do not know about these harmful ingredients. In order to be fresh, clean, and fragrant, we search for the best-branded hair care products. Believing more in perfecting our appearance, we do not pay heed to what are we using for hair care. Nevertheless, we should not be careless. For this carelessness, can cause harm to our health. Therefore, we should learn as much as we can about the

chemicals used in commercial shampoos and read the shampoo bottle labels carefully, rather

than rely more on the false promises made by the shampoo manufactures.

Benefits of Herbal Shampoo

Benefits of Making Your Own Herbal Shampoo and Hair Treatments

Eating the right kinds of food, drinking a lot of water, and getting enough rest are some of the factors that can make your hair beautiful and healthy. Shampoos and hair conditioners are also essential for keeping it well nourished and clean. However, you should know that many hair treatment products available in the market, including those that are said to be 100% natural, contain synthetic fragrances, petrochemicals, detergents and some allergens. Without you knowing it, the harsh ingredients present in these hair care products actually strip your hair of natural oils. That is why the popularity of homemade herbal shampoos and hair treatments is increasing.

Contrary to what most people think, you do not actually need to buy the latest shampoo and spend a fortune to have beautiful-looking hair. You can create your own all-natural herbal shampoo and hair treatments in the comfort of your own home and have great-looking hair. Homemade herbal shampoos and hair treatments do not contain the chemicals and synthetic ingredients used in commercial hair products so it is safe to use them daily. These products contain pure ingredients that you can even find from your own garden or botanical stores. They are not only natural but also inexpensive. They are gentle to your scalp and constantly nourish your hair.

Nowadays, more people are beginning to love the idea of making their own all-natural herbal shampoo and hair treatments for the many benefits they can get from these products. Here are some of those benefits:

Free of Toxins

The main ingredients in commercial shampoos are SLES (sodium laureth sulfate) and SLS (sodium lauryl sulfate). These are known as surfactants and they are used to wash out the dirt and sebum on your hair. These are toxic chemicals and can cause skin irritations. What is healthy about using herbal shampoos is that they are all created with the use of natural ingredients such as essential oils, herbs, spices, and water, so you are sure you are not using toxins to wash your hair.

Fresh Ingredients

Since you are creating homemade herbal hair treatments with the use of natural ingredients that you have just bought from a botanical store or picked right from your own garden, you know that you are using fresh ingredients that can produce results that are more effective. Store-bought shampoos and hair treatments were prepared many months prior to your purchase. This means that the ingredients used in the product are no longer fresh or might have already decayed or expired. In this case, aside from losing its benefits, such product is no longer safe to use, as it can be harmful as well.

Custom-made

What is good about preparing your own natural herbal shampoo and hair treatments is that you can choose your favorite ingredients. You can experiment on the ingredients as well. You can either add more or remove some of these ingredients, depending on what ingredients work for you or are compatible with your hair type. For instance, if your hair is too oily, you can choose lemon, chamomile, rosemary or any essential oils that are good for oily hair. You can pick peppermint, lemon balm, bay leaf, or any herbs that are perfect for oily hair. If after trying many different shampoos you notice that your dandruff keeps coming back, you can try adding apple cider vinegar into your new shampoo solution and see for yourself.

Cost-saving

You can save a lot by creating your own natural hair products. There are actually good shampoos and hair conditioners that can provide the same benefits as the ones you can make. These products are also made of organic and all-natural ingredients and do not contain harmful ingredients, but they can cost a lot. In addition, you can see many low-cost hair products on the shelves, but they usually contain the harmful chemicals and artificial ingredients. However, when you decide to buy the ingredients to make your own natural shampoo and hair treatments, you can get the most benefit because you know you will be using safe ingredients and getting the most out of your money.

Fun

Using your creativity to create something useful can bring joy and fulfillment and this is also true for creating your own natural hair treatment products. You can try new ingredients each time until you come up with the one that you like best. You will be surprised to discover that soon enough you want to make a new one to see any difference in the results or to check which works best for you. Whenever you try to use different ingredients, you get more curious and excited. Sooner or later you will not only want to create one for yourself alone but also for your friends or family. It is even more fun if you can spend some time with your friends or family to create your special herbal shampoos. What's more, this can develop into a new hobby or a new business venture.

Shampoo Base Ingredients

When making your own homemade hair products be sure to keep them in clean containers and store them in a cool, dry location. Also, make sure that you wash your hands properly before, during, and after using homemade hair care products so as to avoid germ cross-contamination. If you find that, your homemade shampoo has started to separate, simply give the mixture a vigorous stir. However, if it starts to smell a little funny – then it probably has gone bad and it is high time to throw it out.

Basic Herbal Shampoo Ingredients

Herbal shampoos only require very few ingredients:

- **Distilled Water**

Unfortunately, regular tap or faucet water, and even so-called purified water, contains minerals and other kinds of impurities. These minerals and impurities can actually leave harsh mineral deposits that build up over time on your hair. This can make your hair appear greasy and dull. Distilled water is simply water from which such minerals and impurities have been successfully removed through distillation. Distilled water is widely used in a variety of settings due to the fact that is leaves less mineral deposits. Although it is never suggested to actually drink distilled water, it can be used perfectly for homemade herbal shampoos and treatments.

- **Castile Soap**

This soap is comprised primarily of vegetable oils, such as jojoba, hemp, coconut, and olive oils. Castile soap can be bought in either liquid or flake form. However, in its most purest form, Castile soaps are created using only virgin olive oil. If you are able to find pure olive oil Castile soap, then this is the best type to use in your homemade herbal shampoos and other hair treatments. Unlike other soaps that are made from animal fat, Castile soap is non-toxic and biodegradable, which means that it does not harm the environment in any way. One of the best brands to purchase is Dr. Bronner's Castile soap – it is available online and at various health shops. You can purchase it in an unscented formula, as well as in Almond, Peppermint, and other such refreshing scents. Castile soap can be used as a general household cleanser, pet shampoo, shaving foam, baby care, and, of course, for hair and body cleansing.

- **Herbs and Essential Oils**

There is an abundance of essential oils and natural herbs from which to choose when creating your own herbal shampoo and hair treatment. Regardless of the recipe you to choose to replicate, you will always need to soak your herbs and oils into the distilled water first. This will allow the nutrients and scents from the herbs and oils to better infuse your shampoo. Think of it as simply making a cup of tea – first you steep the herbs in the water, and then you strain the tea so as to leave the tea leaves behind. Whether you decide to use essential oils, fresh herbs, or dried herbs will depend on the herb itself.

Some of the most commonly used herbs and oils are:

- Lavender
- Rosemary
- Rose petals
- Chamomile
- Nettle
- Peppermint
- Lemon
- Lemon grass
- Clary Sage

Shampoo Base Recipes

Here are a few homemade shampoo base recipes:

- **2 Ingredients Natural Shampoo Recipe**

- 1 cup water
- 1 tablespoon baking soda

1. Mix the ingredients into a clean empty shampoo bottle.
2. Shake gently before using.

- **Natural Shampoo Base Recipe**

- 3 oz. liquid Castile Soap
- 8 oz. water
- ¼ teaspoon olive oil

1. Place water in a clean empty bottle. Add oil and Castile soap.
2. Shake well before using.

- **Natural Shampoo Base Recipe with Coconut Milk**

- 1/3 cup liquid Castile soap
- ¼ cup homemade coconut milk
- 20 drops lavender oil

1. Place all ingredients in an empty and clean used shampoo bottle.

2. Shake well before every use.

- **Basic Shampoo Formula**

- 2 tablespoons of liquid Castile soap
- 1 cup of spring or distilled water
- 2 tablespoons of dried herbs of your choice or ¼ cup fresh herbs of your choice
- 1 teaspoon apricot kernel oil or almond oil
- 2 drops of essential oil of your choice

1. In a clean 10-ounce glass jar, place the fresh or dried herbs. Make sure that the glass jar has a lid that closes properly.

2. Boil the spring or distilled water and then pour the water gently over the herbs in the glass jar.

3. Close the lid and let the mixture steep for at least 10 to 20 minutes.

4. Next, strain the water from the herb infusion into a separate bowl.

5. Slowly add in the liquid Castile soap, as well as the almond oil or the apricot kernel oil and mix thoroughly.

6. Add in the essential oil to scent and continue mixing.

7. Place the mixture into a plastic container, or reuse an empty shampoo bottle.

Herbal Infusions

Choose herbs for your shampoo that will enhance your hair color and texture, and that address any special needs you may have. You can mix and match herbs from the following lists to develop an individualized combination that is best for your hair.

Dry: Elder flowers, comfrey root, avocado, orange blossoms

Normal: Horsetail, clover, dandelion

Oily: Lemon grass, strawberry leaf, watercress, white willow bark

Ethnic: Olive oil, comfrey, cherry bark, nettle

Shine: Vinegar, raspberry, egg, nettle, quassia

Manageability: Yogurt, beer, cherry bark

Softness: Marjoram, cherry bark, olive oil, burdock root

Dandruff: Peppermint, comfrey, white willow bark, birch bark, nettle, vinegar

Growth: Rosemary, St. John's Wort, sage, nettle, basil, onion juice

Herbal Infusion Natural Shampoo Recipes

Custom-made shampoos are not as thick or as quickly washed out as commercially acquired mixtures; however, they will successfully clean hair with naturally sustaining elements and botanicals. Since homemade herbal shampoos are so much gentler, you can expect that your hair will not feel as squeaky-clean in the wake of washing. This is because it will not be stripped of its natural oils, as it would be with commercial shampoo!

- **Herbal Shampoo Recipe**

- 8 ounces (1 cup) of water
- 3 oz. Liquid Castile Soap
- 1-2 TBSP dried natural herbs of your choice
- 20-60 drops of essential oil of your choice
- 1/4 tsp natural Jojoba or Olive oil (adjust as needed - utilize more for dry hair or less if your hair is naturally sleek)

1. Make a homegrown imbuement by spilling bubbling water over the herbs.
2. Cover the mixture, and permit them to soak for no less than 4 hours.
3. Strain the herbs out and put the saved fluid into a jug.
4. Then include the Castile cleanser and oils. Your homegrown cleanser is presently prepared to utilize.
5. Continuously shake well before use since the substance will regularly separate.

- **Homemade Herbal Shampoo Using Distilled Water**

- 8 oz. (1 cup) of distilled water
- 2 teaspoons of dried Rosemary
- 2 teaspoons of dried Rose Petals
- 3 ounces liquid Castile soap
- 3 Tablespoon Aloe Vera Gel
- ¼ teaspoon of Jojoba Oil
- 30 drops of pure Rosemary Essential Oil

1. Place the rosemary and flower petals into a jug.
2. Fill the jug with bubbling water and quickly put a top over the container. Let this mixture soak for at least 30 minutes.
3. Strain the herbs.
4. Let the remaining liquid cool to room temperature.
5. Place the liquid into a clean recycled shampoo container. (You can purchase another bottle like a flask or other kind of bottle)
6. Add the Castile cleanser to the compartment. Then add the Jojoba Oil and essential oil.
7. Finally add the Aloe Vera Gel.
8. Shake well! You now have your very own natural hand crafted shampoo. You will need to shake this mixture before you utilize it.

This cleanser ought to keep going for a few weeks. In the event that it will take you longer than that to utilize the entire substance, you may want to think about keeping some of it in the refrigerator to extend its lifespan.

- **Shimmer & Shine Shampoo**

• 1/2 mug water

• 2 tablespoons dried, or 1/3 mug fresh Chamomile, Lavender or Rosemary

• 1/2 mug of the Basic Shampoo

• 2 tablespoons glycerin

1. Combine the water and herbs together and heat gently to make a solid tea.
2. Let the mixture soak for no less than 20 minutes.
3. Add in the Basic Shampoo and the glycerin to the water mixture and blend well.
4. Put the mixture into a clean bottle, flask, or jug.
5. Let the mixture sit overnight to thicken.
6. To utilize: Shampoo and rinse well.

- **Homemade Herbal Shampoo**

- ½ cup of Castile cleanser with any scent that you prefer, such as Peppermint, or Eucalyptus

- 1 Tablespoon of Rosemary – animates the hair follicles and serves to avoid untimely hairlessness

- 1 Tablespoon of Sage – has cell reinforcements and increases the life of the shampoo and is also antibacterial

- 1 Tablespoon of Brambles – goes about as a blood purifier, blood stimulator, holds a huge wellspring of supplements for hair development

- 1 Tablespoon of Lavender – controls the creation of sebaceous organic oil and decreases irritated and flaky scalp conditions

- 2000 mg of MSM – gives natural sulfur to your scalp, which enhances the wellbeing and quality of your hair. It likewise serves to drive natural supplementation into the skin and hair follicles where they can do the most great
- One clean 8 oz. plastic bottle or flask, or any viable shampoo container

1. Blend the herbs in a jug or container that has a lid.
2. Heat up 2 mugs of refined water. Include three stacking tablespoons of the blended herbs into the bubbling water.
3. Pull the bubbling water and herbs off the stove. Let the herb mixture sit for 30 – 40 minutes.
4. Put the 2000mg of MSM into the herb mixture following the 30 minutes of cooling.
5. Once the MSM is softened, or 40 minutes has passed – whichever is sooner, strain the mixture into a dish.
6. Pour 2 to 2 1/2 oz. of the strained natural tea into the 8 oz. plastic container.
7. Next, pour 4 oz. of Castile cleanser into the 8 oz. plastic container. Top the container and shake well to blend the elements together.
8. The shampoo is now ready for use.

- **Natural Herbal Shampoo for Oily Hair**

- 1 cup of distilled water
- 2 teaspoons of dried Rosemary
- 2 teaspoons of dried Rose Petals
- 3/8 cup of liquid Castile soap
- 3 Tablespoons of Aloe Vera Gel
- ¼ teaspoon of Jojoba Oil
- 30 drops of pure Rosemary Essential Oil

1. Place the Rose Petals and the Rosemary into a jug.
2. Fill the jug with bubbling water and quickly put a top over the container. Let this mixture soak for at least 30 minutes.
3. Strain the herbs.
4. Let the liquid cool down to room temperature.
5. Place the liquid into a clean recycled shampoo container or other such bottle.
6. Add the Castile cleanser to the bottle before adding in the Jojoba Oil, essential oil, and the Aloe Vera Gel.
7. Shake well. You now have your very own natural hand crafted shampoo. You will need to shake this mixture before you utilize it.

This cleanser ought to keep going for a few weeks. In the event that it will take you longer than that to utilize the entire substance, you may want to think about keeping some of it in the refrigerator to extend its lifespan.

- **Natural Herbal Shampoo for Dry Hair**

- ¼ cup Aloe Vera gel
- ¼ cup liquid Castile soap
- ¼ cup distilled water
- ¼ teaspoon Jojoba Oil
- 1 teaspoon glycerin

1. Combine all ingredients in a clean empty bottle. Mix well to combine.
2. Shake before using.

- **Natural Herbal Shampoo for Flaky Scalp**

- ¼ cup liquid Castile soap
- ¼ cup distilled water
- 6 very finely ground Cloves
- 3 tablespoons Apple Juice
- 1 tablespoon Apple Cider Vinegar
- ½ teaspoon Jojoba Oil

1. Place all ingredients in a small grinder. Grind on low for half a minute.
2. Wet your hair with warm water. Use the mixture to shampoo your hair and scalp. Rinse.

- **Natural Herbal Shampoo for Shiny Hair**

- ¼ cup liquid lemon Castile soap
- ¼ cup distilled water
- 2 tablespoons Sweet Almond Oil
- 2 tablespoons dried Rosemary
- ¼ teaspoon your choice of essential oil

1. Bring distilled water to a boil. Steep the Rosemary until fragrant.
2. Strain the leaves and allow it to cool for a while.
3. Mix all the remaining ingredients. Add it to the water. Stir well.
4. Pour in an empty and clean bottle.
5. Shake well before using.

- **Natural Herbal Shampoo for Soothing and Calming Hair**

- 6 Chamomile tea bags

- 1 cup lavender Castile soap
- 1 cup distilled water
- 1 ½ tablespoons glycerin

1. Boil 1 cup of water. Steep the chamomile teabags for 20 minutes. Discard the teabags.
2. Add the Castile soap. Add glycerin. Stir until blended well.
3. Pour in an empty and clean bottle with lid.

Natural Herbal Shampoo for Sensitive Scalp

- 20 drops Sage oil
- ¼ cup Castile soap
- 1 cup boiling water
- 2 tablespoons Peppermint
- ½ teaspoon Grapeseed Oil

1. Place boiling water in a bowl. Add the herbs. Cover and leave for a few hours.
2. Strain the herbs. Add and gently mix all the ingredients. Pour mixture in a squeeze bottle.
3. Allow it to sit for a few hours before using.

Natural Shampoo to Lighten and Freshen up Blonde Hair

- 6 chamomile tea bags
- 1 cup distilled water
- ¼ cup Castile soap
- 1 teaspoon glycerin

1. Bring water to boil. Steep teabags for 20 minutes. Discard teabags.

2. Add the Castile soap. Mix. Add glycerin and mix it well.

3. Pour in an empty and clean bottle with seal.

- **Natural Shampoo for Alopecia**

- 100 ml of the natural base shampoo
- 8 drops Carrot essential oil
- 15 drops Jojoba essential oil
- 2 drops Tea Tree oil
- 7 drops Lavender essential oil
- 7 drops Rosemary essential oil

1. Place all the ingredients in a bowl. Stir well to combine.

2. Store in an empty and clean container with lid.

3. Use as a regular shampoo.

- **Natural Shampoo for Greasy Hair**

- ¼ cup natural base shampoo (recipe on the first page)
- ½ cup boiled water
- 2 tablespoons chopped fresh Mint
- 1 tablespoon Rosemary

1. Place boiled water in a bowl. Add Rosemary and Mint. Mix.

2. Add the natural base shampoo. Mix and allow the mixture to steep for at least 30 minutes.

3. Strain and pour into a clean and empty jar.

4. Use as a shampoo.

- **Natural Shampoo for Babies**

- ¼ cup warm water
- ¼ cup unscented Castile mild baby soap
- ¼ cup Avocado oil
- 4 drops Lavender essential oil

1. Place all the ingredients in an empty and clean container with lid.
2. Shake to combine.
3. Shake well every before using.
4. Take extra caution as the Castile soap is not tear-free.

Natural Shampoos with Essential Oil Recipes

- **Natural Shampoo with Essential Oil for Yummy Smelling Hair**

- 25 drops Lemon Grass Essential Oil
- 15 drops Lavender Essential Oil
- 10 drops Lemon Essential Oil
- ¼ cup Coconut Milk
- ¼ cup Honey
- ½ cup liquid Castile soap
- 1 tablespoon Vitamin E oil
- 2 tablespoons Coconut oil

1. Place all the ingredients in an empty and clean container. Place the lid on. Shake gently to combine.
2. Shake before using.

- **Natural Shampoo with Essential Oil for Fragile Hair**

- 20 drops Clary Sage Essential Oil
- 15 drops Wild Orange Essential Oil
- 15 drops Lavender Essential Oil
- ¼ cup Honey
- ¼ cup Coconut Milk
- 2 tablespoons Coconut Oil
- 1 tablespoon Vitamin E oil

1. Place all the ingredients in an empty and clean container. Place the lid on. Shake gently to combine.
2. Shake before use.

Hair Spritz Recipes

- **Rosemary Spritz**

- 2 Rosemary teabags
- 10 oz. water
- 4 drops Ylang Ylang oil
- 5 drops Tea Tree oil

1. Prepare a clean spritz bottle.
2. Bring the water to a boil. Turn off heat.
3. Steep the tea bags for 1 hour. Pour the water into prepared bottle. Add both the oil.
4. Shake well and use.
5. Place in the fridge to extend lifespan.

- **Aloe Vera Spritz**

- 2 parts Aloe Vera juice
- 4 parts water
- 2 parts glycerin
- 1 part Olive oil
- 1 part Coconut oil
- A few drops of your favorite essential oil

1. Combine and mix well all the ingredients in an empty and clean spritz bottle.
2. Place the homemade spritz in the fridge to extend the lifespan.

Hair Mask Recipes

- **Strawberry Natural Hair Mask**

- 1 cup a little mushy texture Strawberries
- 2 tablespoons Olive oil
- 1 egg yolk

1. Mix up all the ingredients well until the strawberries looks like a juice.
2. Massage mixture onto hair and leave for 20 minutes.
3. Rinse using a mild shampoo.

- **Green Tea Natural Hair Mask**

- 2 tablespoons strong fresh Green Tea
- 1 egg yolk
- 1 tablespoon mustard powder

1. Combine all ingredients in a bowl.
2. Mix until you will teach a creamy consistency. You may add more green tea if your mask mixture is too thick.
3. Apply mixture onto hair. Put on shower cap and leave for 25 minutes. Rinse.
4. Shampoo and condition hair as normal.

Oil Treatment Recipes

Oil medicines are an extraordinary approach to condition, sooth, cleans, purify, and strengthen the hair and scalp. Leaving hair delicate, glossy, and sleek, they are superb for treating harmed, dry, dull, or bunched up hair and scalp conditions. A couple of drops of either of these formulas can additionally be utilized to better manage those dry or wild-looking locks!

To utilize, put a little oil into your palm and rub it deep into your scalp and hair, making sure to cover your roots evenly. Leave in for no less than 30 minutes. However, the longer you can leave it, the better. Try wrapping your hair in a turbie or shower cap and leave the oil until just before bedtime when you can wash it all out. Make sure that you wash out all of the oil completely. Do not worry if your hair feels a bit slick after washing it - it ought to ingest the remaining oil as it dries. High temperature delays the oil's entrance into the hair shaft, improving its benefits. Harness the power of the sun, by sitting in direct sunlight, or by a wood stove, chimney, or even in a sauna.

You can also treat yourself to a hot oil medication by tenderly warming the oil to 100 degrees Fahrenheit and then rubbing it into your hair and scalp with your fingers. Pull your hair back, and wrap it up in a plastic shower cap, and lastly wrap it up with a thick cotton or microfiber towel to help hold in as much heat as possible. Leave it on your head for at least 60 minutes, and then wash it all out thoroughly.

- **Fundamental Hair Oil Treatment Recipe**

- ¼ cup Jojoba or Olive Oil
- 10 – 30 drops of an essential oil of your choosing

1. To make, essentially mix together the Jojoba or Olive Oils into a jug and then include the drops of essential oil.
2. Shake well before each use so as to thoroughly mix the oils together.

- **Homemade Infused Hair Oil**

- 1 cup of Olive Oil or Jojoba Oil
- 3 Tablespoons of dried herbs of your choice

1. In a glass container, mix together the Olive Oil or Jojoba Oil with the dried herbs.
2. Close the lid tightly and allow to imbue for three to six weeks.
3. Shake the container ever day during this time frame.
4. When the time is up, strain the herbs from imbued oil.
5. When stored in a cool, dry spot, the imbued oil should last for at least on year.

- **Rosemary Herbal Oil**

This adaptable oil has numerous uses; as a rub for arthritis, pain, and gout. It can also be used to treat scalp issues such as dandruff and other irritations. To use a hot oil treatment for damaged hair: Warm the oil carefully, and then tenderly rub a little bit into the scalp and hair, wrap a towel around your head, and leave on for at least one hour.

- 8 oz. of Extra-Virgin Olive Oil
- 1/2 cup of fresh Rosemary

The best system for making Rosemary oil is to utilize a slow cooker; however, you can also prepare the oil using your stovetop as well.

Unless you are unsure as to whether or not the plant from which you picked the Rosemary was treated with any pesticides, it is best not to wash the Rosemary. At the same time, on the off chance that you do wash the sprig of Rosemary, make certain that it completely dry before using it to make the oil.

It is not important to strip the leaves from the rosemary plant; instead, you should delicately squash the sprigs by tenderly rubbing them between your clean hands. This starts to discharge the grand aroma of the herb.

- **Stovetop Rosemary Oil**

Utilize a substantial pot that heats up evenly. Avoid using any non-enameled cast iron or aluminum pots. Once you have placed the crushed Rosemary into the pot, you can gently pour in the oil. Place on low heat for about 5 - 10 minutes. You need the oil to warm however, not simmer.

Turn the heat off and allow the Rosemary to permeate the oil for at least an hour. Strain the mixture into a clean, dry glass container. Close the container tightly and store away from any direct sunlight or heat, preferably in a cupboard where it can sit, undisturbed, at room temperature for 2 months. Alternatively, you can place the container in your refrigerator for up to 6 months.

- **Making Rosemary Oil in a Slow Cooker**

Set the fresh Rosemary into your slow cooker and then cover it with the oil. For one hour, allow the mixture to cook on the high setting.

After an hour has passed, you can then turn off your slow cooker and allow the oil to come down to room temperature. Strain the oil into clean and dry glass container and cover tightly. Store the oil away from direct sunlight or heat and allow it to sit at room temperature for at least 2 months. Or place it in your refrigerator for up to 6 months.

- **Homemade Ayurveda Oil**

- 1 Tablespoon of Neem oil
- 1 Tablespoon of Castor oil
- 4 Tablespoons of Sesame oil
- 2 Tablespoons of Sweet Almond oil
- 2 Tablespoons of Virgin Coconut oil
- 5 Tablespoons of Water

- 1 Tablespoon of powdered Amla berry seeds
- 1 Tablespoon of ground Fenugreek leaves
- 1 Tablespoon of ground Red Hibiscus leaves and petals
- 1 Tablespoon of ground and dried Bhangra leaves
- 1 Tablespoon of ground and dried Brahmi leaves

(You can substitutes the Brahmi leaves with 1 tablespoon of Indian Pennywort or Gotu Kola)

1. Mix all of the dried herbs together in a large heavy bottom pot
2. In a different pot, heat up the water to the point of boiling
3. Pour the boiling water over the dried herbs
4. Allow the herbs to soak in the water for two hours
5. Pour the oil over the hydrated herbs and mix together well
6. Turn the temperature to low and allow the oil to warm slowly
7. Allow to steep, un-covered, on the low heat for an additional 2 to 3 hours
8. Turn off the heat and allow the mixture to cool completely
9. Strain the mixture so as to remove any solids
10. Place the mixture back over the low heat to remove any excess moisture for an additional 30 minutes
11. Once the moisture has evaporated after the 30 minutes, allow the oil to cool before pouring it into a plastic or glass container and storing in a cool, dry location

The oil should be applied right before bed, so that it can infuse with your hair and scalp overnight. In the morning, you can wash and dry your hair as normal. If you have normal hair, then you should use this oil at least once a week; however, if your hair is dry, you should use the oil at least twice a week. However, if you have oily hair, you should only use this oil once every two weeks. Prior to application, make sure that the oil is either warm to the touch or is at room temperature.

Apply the oil by separating your hair and spreading the oil with your fingers along your scalp. Continue until your entire scalp has been covered with the oil. Never pour the oil directly onto your scalp.

With your fingertips, massage your scalp in a circular motion for 30 minutes to help stimulate blood flow. Next, if you have split ends, gently rub the oil into the ends of your hair. Remember to put a soft towel over your pillow before going to bed to protect your bedding from the oil. Feel free to wash and dry your hair as normal in the morning.

- **Coconut Oil Hair Treatment**

- 2 cups of Coconut oil
- 10 gm Hibiscus petals
- 5 gm of Fenugreek seeds
- 5 gm of Curry leaves
- 5 gm of Neem leaves

1. Heat the Coconut oil. Once it starts to boil, slowly add in the hibiscus petals, and then include the Fenugreek seeds, Curry leaves, and the Neem leaves as well.
2. Allow the mixture to cool.
3. Once cooled, pour the mixture into a glass container.
4. Store it in a cool, dry location for several weeks.
5. Strain the mixture again into another clean glass container. It is now ready to be used.

- **Natural Hot Oil with Black Tea**

- 1cup Sweet Almond oil
- 3 drops Chamomile oil
- Black tea

1.	Place the Sweet Almond oil and leaves of the black tea in a small bowl. Place it on a larger bowl with very hot water to warm it.

2.	Strain using cheesecloth and place the strained oil in a bowl.

3.	Add the Chamomile oil. Stir.

4.	Separate your hair into4 part, 2 down and 2 up. Using a pastry brush, apply hot oil to the bottom part first. Massage hot oil into your scalp.

5.	Wrap your hair with a plastic wrap followed by a hot towel and leave for half an hour.

6.	To rinse off oil, shampoo your hair at least twice.

- **Natural Hot Oil for Normal Hair**

- 1 cup virgin Coconut oil
- 2 tablespoon Avocado oil
- 2 tablespoon Safflower oil
- 1 tablespoon Jojoba oil

1.	Place the oil in a measuring cup glass. Heat it in the microwave for 2 minutes.

2.	Place the warmed oil in an applicator bottle to make it easier to apply onto hair.

3.	Soak you hair with water for 5 minutes. Evenly dispense oil into your hair with your hands. Massage from your scalp to the ends. Cover hair with a plastic cap. Process under a hooded dryer for 20 minutes. A steamer will work as well.

4.   Remove the plastic cap. Shampoo and condition as usual.

Herbal Hair Rinses

Hair rinses are very simple and easy to make, and they are commonly used to condition both the hair and the scalp. They smooth the hair and add volume and shine. They also help to improve the hair's natural highlights.

- **Basic Herbal Hair Rinse**

- 3 Tablespoon of dried herbs of your choice
- 2 Cups of distilled water

1. Bring the water to slow boil.
2. Pour the boiling water over the dried herbs.
3. Allow the mixture to infuse overnight – or at least for eight hours.
4. Use a sieve and separate the herbs from the water.
5. Pour the water mixture into a glass container to store in a cool, dry place.

However, it is best if the herb rinse is used within a few hours of concoction. Apply the rinse by slowly pouring it over your hair, making sure to massage it gently into the scalp and roots of your hair. It is best if you hold your hair over a huge bowl or sink in order to catch any excess liquid. You can then use this liquid to reapply to your head again. Once all the liquid has been applied, you can either wash it out completely, or allow the mixture to dry first.

- **Natural Vinegar Rinse**

  - 3 Tablespoon of dried herbs of your choice
  - 1 Cup of Apple Cider Vinegar

1. Mix together the herbs and the Apple Cider Vinegar in a glass container with a lid.
2. Allow the mixture to infuse together for three to six weeks.
3. Each day during this time period, shake the container to mix up the contents.
4. When the time is up, strain out the dried herbs.
5. Pour the remaining vinegar mixture into another clean container.

To use this as a rinse, apply one to two tablespoons to your hair. Massage the vinegar liquid into your scalp and hair, making sure to cover the roots and the ends. Rinse out thoroughly.

- **Organic Vinegar Rinse**

  - 1 Cup of water
  - 1 Tablespoon of organic vinegar

1. Mix together the water and organic vinegar in a glass container.
2. Apply the rinse as directed above.

Vinegar rinses contain the exact same benefits as regular water-based rinses; but they have the added benefit of being able to restore your hair's natural pH balance. When mixed properly and stored in a cool, dry location, vinegar rinses can last up to one year.

Vinegar rinses are perfect for treating dandruff and other scalp irritations, as well as treating oil hair.

- **Lavender Rosemary Softening Hair Rinse**

- 3 Tablespoons of Apple Cider Vinegar
- 4 Cups of water
- 1 teaspoon of borax
- 1/2 cup of dried Lavender
- 1/2 cup of dried Rosemary

1. In a large pot, bring the water to a quick boil.
2. When the water is at rolling boil, remove the pot from the stove and stir in the Apple Cider vinegar and the borax.
3. Stir in the Lavender and Rosemary and mix until the herbs are saturated.
4. Allow the mixture to sit for two to four hours or longer – the longer it sits, the stronger the rinse will become.
5. Once the mixture turns to a caramel brownish color, drain the herbs from the liquid and pour the remaining liquid into a clean glass container.
6. Allow the mixture to steep overnight before using.
6. Keep the mixture in the refrigerator until ready to use.

This rinse can be used either alone, or after you have shampooed and conditioned your hair as normal. Simply pour the rinse over your hair, making sure to saturate it completely. Next, use fresh, warm water to rinse the Lavender, Rosemary, and Apple Cider Vinegar from your hair.

One caveat here, since the Lavender, Rosemary, and Apple Cider Vinegar Rinse resembles a cup of brewed tea, its natural coloring may stain your towels – so be sure to use a dark colored one to dry your hair, or at least one that you do no mind staining. If you wanted, you could simply leave the Lavender, Rosemary, and Apple Cider Vinegar in your hair and dry per usual.

- **Natural Lavender-Mint Hair Rinse For All Hair Types**

- 1 cup boiling water
- ½ cup Apple Cider Vinegar
- ½ tablespoon dried Lavender leaves
- 1 tablespoon dried Mint leaves

1. Place the dried mint and lavender leaves in a bowl. Add vinegar. Pour boiling water over.
2. Allow the mixture to completely cool. Strain.
3. Apply the mixture to your scalp as a final rinse after your shampoo.
4. Rinse your hair well with the coldest water you can stand.

- **Natural Sage Hair Rinse for Brunette Hair**

- ¼ cup fresh Sage leaves
- 2 cups water

1. Place sage leaves in a bowl.
2. Boil water and pour it over the sage leaves. Allow it to cool.
3. Strain.
4. Pour it over your clean hair for a final rinse.

5. Do not rinse it with water.

- **Natural Chamomile-Rhubarb Hair Rinse for Blonde Hair**

- ¼ cup chopped rhubarb stalks
- 2 tablespoons dried chamomile flowers
- 2 cups water

1. Place all the ingredients in a saucepan. Heat it gently until boiling. Turn off heat.
2. Allow the mixture to steep until cool. Strain the solids off.
3. Massage the hair rinse mixture onto your clean and damp hair.
4. Do not rinse your hair with water.

- **Natural Hibiscus Hair Rinse for Redheads**

- ¼ cup fresh Hibiscus flower
- 2 cups water

1. Bring water to boil. Pour it over the Hibiscus flower.
2. Allow it to steep until cool.
3. Strain solids.
4. Pour the rinse mixture over your clean hair.
5. Do not rinse it out with water.

Natural Dry Shampoo Recipes

- **Natural Dry Shampoo for Dark Hair**

- ½ tablespoon Cocoa powder
- 5 drops Lavender essential oil
- 1 tablespoon baking soda
- 1 tablespoon cornstarch

1. Place all ingredients in a bowl. Mix.
2. Pat a brush with the mixture to your hair from the roots. Let it sit for a few minutes. Hands shake it and brush out lightly.

- **Natural Dry Shampoo for Normal Hair**

- 10 drops Lemon essential oil
- 2 tablespoons rice flour
- 2 tablespoons corn starch
- 2 tablespoons Arrowroot powder

1. Combine all ingredients and mix well.
2. Pat a brush with the mixture to your hair from the roots.
3. Allow it to sit for a few minutes.
4. Hands shake it and brush out lightly.

Summary

Achieving hair that is shiny, smooth, and full of bounce without abusing it with an abundance of synthetic chemicals is not hard. Neither is it expensive. You do not need fancy contraptions, or exotic sounding ingredients that only grow on far-away islands in order to make your own homemade herbal shampoos and other hair treatments.

In fact, you can create your own magical hair shampoo and hair treatments just using common equipment that is found in every kitchen. Even the ingredients themselves are usually stocked in kitchen pantries as well, such as Apple Cider Vinegar and Rosemary. Other specialty herbs, oils, and flowers can be purchased easily either online or at your local health food store.

In this book, you will learn the following:

- The History of Shampoos

- Why commercial shampoos are actually bad for your hair

- What cancer-causing ingredients are in your shampoo right now

- How to read the label of your shampoo bottle

- Which chemicals are actually good for your hair

- Learn the benefits of creating your own herbal shampoo

- Find out which common household tools to use to create your own herbal shampoos

- Learn which natural ingredients - that are already in your pantry - you can use to create your own herbal shampoos

- Discover which herbs, oils, and flowers are best suited for your hair type and condition

- Recipes for Herbal Shampoos, Hair Spritzes, Oil Treatments, Hairs Masks, Hair Rinses, and Herbal Dry Shampoos

Knowing which common kitchen utensils and ingredients, along with knowing the best herbs, oils, and flowers to use for your hair's specific needs, can go a long way in helping you create delightful herbal shampoos and treatments at home.

The time you invest today in learning about these recipes, as well as in creating these formulas, will reward you with hair that is radiant and healthy for years to come.